Gastric Band Hypnosis: Beginners Guided & Self-Hypnosis For Weight Loss, Burning Fat, Overcoming Food Addiction, Eating Healthy Including Positive Affirmations & Meditations

By Meditation Made Effortless

Table of Contents

To the Narrator

The Introduction, Induction, and Deepener should be 45 Min Long

Hypnotic Gastric Band should be 30 Min long

Eat smaller portions should be 20 Min long

Develop self-love should be 25 Min long

Overcome junk food cravings 30 Min

should be 25 min long

Stop emotional eating should be 15 min long

Ego strengthening script should be 25 min long

More weight loss should be 15 min long

Weight object of the past should be 30 min long

Reinforcement Script should be 20 min long

Affirmations – should be 50 min long

"…" means take a breath while speaking before you continue.

PAUSE (for a few breaths)

LONGER PAUSE (give time to allow the listener time to imagine what you've suggested)

Introduction

Thank you for choosing **Gastric Band Hypnosis audio**...And choosing this audio only means, you have taken a step towards loving yourself even more. In the past, you may have gained weight because of many reasons and you are aware of that. You are also aware that it is important to lose extra weight and have a fitter and healthier body. That is why you are listening to this audio. Isn't it?

Hypnotic gastric band also called as virtual gastric band will allow you to believe that your stomach has shrunk to a size of a golf ball and because of that it can take in smaller amounts of food. You will believe that your stomach is a size of a golf ball and you will eat accordingly exactly how people eat when they get the expensive invasive gastric band surgery done.

Listening to this audio means that you have agreed to believe that your stomach is going to be much smaller in size and that will help you shed extra weight much faster.

When you listen to this recording every day, you reinforce that you are on a weight loss journey where your stomach has shrunken to a size of a golf ball allowing you to eat much lesser, boosting your metabolism, and ultimately helping you lose all the extra weight.

Pause

So, congratulations on taking this step to undergo hypnotic gastric band procedure. Every time you listen to this audio, you get more and more focused on knowing that your stomach has shrunken to a size of a golf ball, you have a band fitted on your stomach, and you eat smaller portions.

Pause

I would like you to sit or lay comfortably, where you will not be distracted. Do not listen to this audio when your mind requires your conscious attention.

Pause

Listen to this audio only when you are relaxed and stationary. Please use headphones so that you can focus on the sound of my voice.

Let us start…

Begin recording

Induction

You are now listening to the sound of my voice… and the sound of my voice only …and as you continue to listen to each word I say…you allow yourself to relax more and more.

Pause

I wonder if you could take a deep breath…hold it for a count of 5… and then exhale.

Pause

Let's start now.

Breathe in Deeply…

Pause

Hold for a count of 5

1... 2...3...4...and 5

Now, exhale...

Pause

Once more, take another deep breath...

Breathe in...

Hold for a count of 5 — 1, 2, 3, 4, 5 (slowly)

Now, breathe out...

Pause

Once more, take another deep breath —

Breathe in

Hold for a count of 5 — 1, 2, 3, 4, 5 (slowly)

Now, breathe out

Pause

And, come back to your normal breathing pattern...

Pause

— And, I wonder... if you could simply bring all your focus and attention to the centre of your eye-brows...with your eyes closed...try to look at the centre of your brows and focus on the point between them...that's right.

Pause

In a moment, I am going to talk to that part of you, which is highly creative...the part that knows exactly how to help you imagine or create anything with the help of your mind's eye.

Pause

And... I know you can do it... because everybody can...we all have a creative mind, that has the ability and capability to create and imagine images in our mind.

I know you must have imagined or visualized or day-dreamed many times in your life. And... our creative part helps us imagine and visualize. Isn't it?

With the help of our creative mind, we can visualize, imagine, write, paint, and dream...and I am going to be talking to that part of you today.

Pause

Deepener

And I wonder if you can imagine or visualize that you are somewhere in a luxury beach resort. And as soon as you enter, you can smell the lovely fragrance at the entrance.

You wonder what scent is that...

The staff caters to your every need and you feel truly pampered and cared for.

In the room of the luxury resort, you notice a beautiful lounger in the patio that overlooks the beautiful sea waters...the lounger has a comfy cushion on it and is perhaps made of sturdy wood. The lounger is tilting a bit backwards for you to relax on it and enjoy the beautiful surroundings. You take a seat and rest your arms on the chair's hand rests.

Pause

You notice the beautiful sun shining and the green tall palm trees swaying with the sea breeze. Far away, you look at the horizon and the many sailboats...perhaps there are 5 or more...

You continue to enjoy the surroundings and enjoy this time alone...so calm and serene.

In a moment, you feel the Sunshine over you and it feels nice and warm...you cover your face with a hat and put the Sun tan lotion all over your body ...and you let yourself soak up the Sun.

Pause

You are all alone here in your room's large patio and there are no people around. You only listen to the sound of the waves and perhaps the sound of the seagulls.

You decide to close your eyes and take a nap...

Pause

And, in a moment, I am going to count you down from 10 down to 0...with each count down, you will be twice as deep and twice as relaxed...

Starting now...

10...relaxing more and more

9...going deeper and deeper

8... into a beautiful state of relaxation

7...allowing yourself to drift down...

5...deeper and deeper...

4...further deep...

3...all your body parts are getting relaxed...

2...even more relaxed...

1...deeper and deeper...

0 – Deep Sleep

Hypnotic Gastric Band Procedure

And as you continue to listen to me...I wonder if you can let go and simply relax your mind and body...for you to easily access your mind's creative part...

A part of you is creative and it allows you to imagine things from the eyes of your mind.

Longer Pause

And I wonder if you can let your creative part help you imagine that you are

entering a door having a long corridor at the end of it -

Somewhere inside your heart...you know that you are entering a procedural room where gastric band procedure will be done. -

Pause

And now slowly and slowly...move towards the door-

You are already aware that this is the safest and renowned place for conducting the procedure -

You trust the doctors and staff...

You already know a lot of people that have lost weight and followed up with the doctors for further consultation here...

You have seen a lot of successful people who have lost so much weight with the help of gastric band, fitted on their stomachs.

Now you must be feeling more confident about this procedure...isn't it?

You believe this will be successful and by the end of the procedure...you stomach would have shrunk to a size of a golf ball.

Longer Pause

The time to enter the clinic is here.

And you push open the door...and enter the clinic...

You are feeling nice about the decision you have made while you enter the clinic

It feels great when you think about the decision taken to go to a procedure involving gastric band

This contracts your stomach...you start feeling full...which in turn results to, you having smaller amounts of food...this way your metabolism increases helping you in losing weight and the ideal goal weight becomes much easier to achieve...

Pause

This is a time of immense happiness for you as today...you have taken a step towards your new version and you have decided to lose weight that has been a a long time desire...isn't it?

Pause

You are now heading towards the procedure room-

You feel relaxed on seeing the staff around you.

You have already booked an appointment with the doctor a week before and you know that the staff is skilled...and they will take good care...

The nurse reminds you that, when they put a silicone band around the stomach...it restricts the food intake which helps in eating less leading you to lose weight easily...

You have a full trust in yourself and the procedure.

Pause

The band will contract it and make it much smaller so that you can take in smaller amounts of foods.

The size would be as small as a golf ball...

It will help in much faster weight loss...

Pause

You will lose weight faster when you consume less food ensuring lesser calorie intake and faster metabolism.

Pause

You might start to think that you are entering a procedural room and that makes you feel calmer and safe...

You are in safe hands...you trust the doctors and nurses...

Pause

As the time passes and the staff talks to you in a friendly way...you feel more and more relaxed...

And in a moment, you notice that you are drifting away into a dream like state while the doctors talk to you about your life...and the sounds of their voices fade away...

You are drifting further and further into a dream like state...a beautiful state of relaxation...and as you enter the deepest state of hypnosis...with your mind's eye...you notice the color of your stomach...

Pause

Perhaps it's either pink or brown...get the knowing of the color of your stomach...

You see it in a particular size...and in a moment...you know that the size of your stomach would reduce when the gastric band will be fitted...

And you are looking forward to the procedure...

You are excited...for this change...the change that will make you feel much better about yourself and much more confident about your body...

Pause

You see that a band is being placed around your stomach...right on top it...making your stomach look really small...

You are closely looking at its size...

And when you observe the size you know that you can only eat much smaller portions of food...

With the gastric band, you can eat food without any diet plans...you only haveto eat smaller portions of healthy and nutritious food...and I know you can do it...because everybody can...

Pause

The band is tightly fitted on the top of your stomach and it stays there for a long time...

You feel much fuller because of the silicone band and you consume food at a slower pace...

The procedure is complete.

Longer Pause

You are free from scars as the procedure has been successfully performed by professional doctors...

Indeed successful...

From now on...your stomach size has been reduced to a size of a golf ball...and it can only accommodate smaller portions of food...that's right...

With this band on your stomach, you will lose weight effortlessly..

Pause

To make the process of digestion faster, you chew food 8 to 12 times...enjoying the flavors of the food...

You are mindful of what you eat and you enjoy each mouthful...

Everyday...you get to feel that your stomach has contracted to the size of a golf ball...and it can take in smaller amounts of food only...

Pause

The procedure is complete...and it has been a success...

You come out of the procedural room...take the discharge slip...the next day...and go back home, feeling absolutely excited for the results that follow...

Imagine being at your goal weight now...

See yourself enjoying what you would enjoy by being at the goal weight...

Longer Pause

I wonder if you can now repeat the following suggestions in your mind after me...

I love consuming smaller portions every day

I feel confident

I make a conscious effort to eat less

I chew my food atleast 8 times

I enjoy the flavors of foods

I relish and enjoy each mouthful...

Eat Smaller Portions

As you continue to listen to each word I say…you allow yourself to stay focused on eating less because you know that your stomach can take in lesser amounts of foods only.

A band is now fitted on the top of your stomach and you can see it with your mind's eye…

The hypnotic gastric band has shrunken the size of your stomach which can now only take lesser amounts of foods…

Listen to this audio more often to know and get convinced that your stomach is much smaller now and with every passing day, you need lesser amounts of food and get satisfied with smaller portions of food…

This will ensure that you reach the goal that you have set for yourself – your ideal body weight…

Note that you must always listen to what my voice is saying. Your mind might wander for a few minutes but you should bring it back by paying attention to this audio...

Pause

You are paying attention to the sound of my voice.

While you pay heed to every word of this recording, you are feeling more relaxed...

As you grasp the word that I say, it is indicating that you are ready to absorb whatever I am saying...

You know now that the size of your stomach is very small...and

You have always wanted to lose weight so your stomach has become smaller helping you to lose weight faster.

Your love for yourself has increased now...

You are aware of what your feelings are, how you behave and act... and the way you think.

Eating a small amount of foods helps in increasing your body metabolism...which in turn results in a faster weight loss.

Every time you eat, you chew food more frequently to get the flavors and taste of the food...

You eat food, enjoy it...and fill your small stomach with nutrients...

Pause

With every word of mine, you start believing how easy it is to intake the right amount of food and lose weight...

And, I would like to talk that creative part of your mind again to show you that you are somewhere in grassy fields...

Longer Pause

The sun is shining bright...

You can smell the smell the fresh air...

Pause

You are in a big magnificent field...

This sunshine is making the field look beautiful and bright...

You feel relaxed as you sit on the ground...

I am wondering if you have ever thought of the reasons why you want to lose weight and get slimmer.

Pause

Are you imagining yourself at your desired weight and size?

Try to get that picture into your mind.

Pause

You are wearing the clothes that you always wanted to wear.

Think of yourself as a person who is much more confident and has high self-esteem.

Pause

How are you feeling about this new weight, what are your body expressions telling you about your new weight and size?

It's time to conceive your actions and your feelings.

You have an inbuilt feeling imbibed in you that makes you realize what is the maximum that you can bear. You will feel that you had sufficient food.

When you get a feeling that you are full, you automatically stop. Sometimes you leave the food on your plate too when you get a feeling that your stomach can't take more.

Pause

It's the time to enter your brain through your imaginative mind.

It is the time to enter your brain, look for a button that signals that your stomach is full.

Start imagining and feel that you are entering your brain.

You are aware that it is your brain that is the governing factor.

It is the time to get inside your brain and look for that particular button

You overeat only when your button does not function well indicating wrong signals, it is the time to get it fixed.

You can only lose weight if the gastric band is in the right place and you are eating less.

You can fix the button so that it functions well and start indicating that the stomach is full.

Pause

The stomach is now of the same size as that of the golf ball.

Longer Pause

You have succeeded in fixing it.

You must check if the button has started working well, indicating the brain that it is the right time to stop eating.

Pause

Now that the button has started functioning giving you the right signals

Start imagining yourself seated in a chair having a table placed in front of you.

The table has a small plate filled with food

Pause

You look towards your plate and eat only that much amount which is ideal for your stomach which has a reduced capacity now

You drink water before eating food

Now you start eating food by gradual chewing and then repeat the step for 15 to 20 times...enjoying the taste and flavours

Pause

Your stomach has reduced in size...so you intake only small amounts of food

Every time you take more food to fill up your plate...you automatically get a signal from the brain and then you stop

That's right

Pause

After you know that you have eaten a lot of food...you just stop

You drink a glass of water after finishing your food...

Every day you feel that your stomach is shrinking and you are getting slimmer by eating small amounts of food...eventually leading to a boost in your metabolism.

You drink at least 8 glasses of water everyday —

Sometimes, you make the water taste good by putting in some lemon or mint...

Every time you eat food, you remember your future image at the target goal weight...

You are aware that if you intake a small amount then you will accomplish your desired goal very soon.

Pause

Every meal boosts up your confidence and energizes you by making you feel confident

From now on...you eat smaller meals...and frequent meals...

Pause

You like small means now (7-8 seconds of pause)

You chew the food atleast 8 to 10 times... (7-8 seconds of pause)

You look ahead for a new to accomplish your goal much sooner (7-8 seconds of pause)

You start feeling grateful about yourself (7-8 seconds of pause)

You stay energized all day by eating small amounts of food (7-8 seconds of pause)

You are much happier and active now (7-8 seconds of pause)

You will be conscious of the amount that you eat from today (7-8 seconds of pause)

You have around 8 glasses of water (7-8 seconds of pause)

Toxins will be released on drinking water and weight loss will be accelerated (7-8 seconds of pause)

You experience faster weight loss (7-8 seconds of pause)

You see a new version of yourself-slimmer, fitter, and happy (7-8 seconds of pause)

You have realized when to stop eating food by sensing how full is your stomach (7-8 seconds of pause)

And as you continue to lose weight and look fitter...I wonder what everyone around you is saying...

Are they proud of what you have achieved?

Longer Pause

Develop Self Love / Inner Child

And I wonder if you can imagine a hallway somewhere...and imagine that hallway leading you to a door...and the door leads you to a garden.

Pause

And, in a moment, you walk towards the door through the hallway...to see how the garden looks like...and it is going to be a beautiful place...

You are now at the door...you touch the door and feel its texture...perhaps its old or new... and in a moment you push open it...

Longer Pause

And as you push open it...you find yourself surrounded by a beautiful garden...

You are in a garden...the garden looks beautiful...and you see many bushes and trees, and feel the lush green grass beneath your feet. As you look around you notice that the garden is magically beautiful with flowers in the bushes...

And as you look further around, you notice a child who looks exactly like how you used to look like when you were young.

Longer Pause

You are amused to see the child and you walk over to the child...the child is sitting on a bench in the garden...

You look at the child and look at the clothes...the shoes...the hair....and the child looks adorable.

You go to the child and give them a big hug...and as that happens the child feels safe and gets into your lap and smiles back.

You tell the child – you are adorable and I love you unconditionally

I love you for who you are and I am proud of you.

You also say that I am sorry for coming to see you after so many years...I am really sorry if I have hurt you ever...I love you and truly do.

Longer Pause

You tell the child that how special he or she is to you...and in a while, you begin to play with the child.

And as you start to play with each other…you begin to enjoy the beautiful bond

That you have with your inner child…its amazing to be in touch with it…isn't it. Together…as you continue to play…you feel and notice that the bond is strengthening…

Pause

And as you both continue to play with each other…the child gets even more comfy with you and comes back in your arms and lap…trusting you even more…

In a moment…you will notice the child integrating into you…and as that happens, you notice…that the child becomes one with you…and you embrace the child…just the way the child is…

Pause

In a moment, as I count from 3 down to 0, with each count down…you notice the child coming closer and then integrating into you…making you whole and complete…as one individual full of self-love...and this only means...that you allow yourself to love even more...

Pause

When it comes to weight loss...you are focused on the path you have chosen to see yourself as fitter, slimmer, and happier....

You are whole and complete...completely focused on achieving your ideal goal weight...and that would be possible if you love yourself completely and unconditionally...

Overcome Junk Food Cravings

And you focus on the sound of my voice and the sound of my voice only...and as you listen to each word I say...you allow yourself to go deeper and deeper and be more and more receptive to what I am saying...

Pause

You know that all your feelings are valid and they are there for a reason. They let you take a certain action so that you are in charge of your life...exactly like how we live in a house and we have electricity, water, power, and kitchen helping us to know what is needed to keep everything going.

Pause

In the same way, our feelings are like electricity, water, power, kitchen, backyard...that allow us to know what is happening to our body and we can take charge of it and take care of ourselves.

Pause

In the same way, by listening to your feelings, you can take care of your body better. If you treat your house the way you have been treating your body...then what would happen?

Perhaps the kitchen groceries would run out of stock if you don't pay attention to the stock or if you do not mow the grass in your backyard or front lawn, you may have overgrown grass and it would perhaps look unkept and ugly...

Longer Pause

And, when you pay attention...you can control everything and take charge of your house.

Similarly, to keep the body working aptly in the best condition, you need to keep attending to the feelings and take actions accordingly for your body's highest good.

If you feel anxious, the action you need to take is to calm yourself down or do a mindful exercise rather than moving towards food and filling yourself up with junk that will make you feel guilty once you have finished eating.

Pause

Another feeling could be stress and it means you have too much on your plate and you are trying to finish everything in a certain amount of time...but instead of turning towards eating junk...you need to look for ways to reduce stress.

Pause

Similarly, you may have many feelings ...but that needs your action to resolve and feel better rather than turning to food and then feel guilty.

From today on, you will be able to pay attention to the feelings and take right actions that allow you to resolve the issue without turning to food.

Longer Pause

You worship your body and in no way you can allow it to get ruined by eating rut or junk food. Junk food is high on sugar and it may give you pleasure temporarily but you know the long-term ill effects of it...isn't it?

And I wonder if you know how eating junk food can affect your cardiovascular health...because they are high in saturated fat, it increases the bad cholesterol in your blood that puts your heart functioning at risk. With too much salt, you may have an increase in high blood pressure, again may put your heart at risk.

Pause

And when it comes to gaining weight, the big culprit is junk food, which is high in calories, sugar, and salt content...and eating junk food three times a week can lead you to gain 1 pound in just about one week.

And, I wonder if you can imagine that you continue to eat junk food for another three months....

Just imagine that now...

Longer Pause

And, you do not have to be like that...you can start the change from today on and instead of junk food, you snack on fruits, vegetables, wheat crackers, fat free dressings and make delicious salads.

You are ready to have a healthy lifestyle with food that is more satisfying than all the rut that you have been eating...

And when any feeling comes, you know how to tackle it exactly how you tackle things at home to keep the home running perfectly...isn't it?

Longer Pause

When you are feeling emotionally or mentally hungry...you divert your thoughts by first showing a "stop signal" to your thought and then distract yourself to resolve the negative feeling in a better way...

And, then when you are physically hungry, you eat healthy food...food that is tasty and healthier...whole grains, lentils, milk, fruits, vegetables...you eat all of this to slim down, look better, and feel amazing...

I know you can do it...because everybody can...

Affirmations

I would like you to now repeat the following in your mind:

- I enjoy eating healthy food
- I am in control of your emotions and actions
- I love myself
- I see myself at my ideal goal weight
- I enjoy eating healthy foods
- I love eating fruits and vegetables and whole grains
- I exercise every day for at least 30 minutes

Stop Emotional Eating

And you continue to focus on the sound of my voice and the sound of my voice only...and this only means you allow yourself to be more receptive to what I am saying...

Your subconscious is very powerful and creative and you will allow your subconscious to show you that a beautiful white light surrounds you from all sides.

You notice the light, perhaps it's the light from the land of the supreme power or whoever you believe in...or perhaps it's your own light of unconditional love and purity...

And it begins to surround you from all sides and enters every part of your body, every cell, fiber, bone and nerve...that's right.

Imagine that happening now...

Longer Pause

And as you continue to feel the lovely white light inside and outside of you...you begin to feel safe...and loved.

That's right...

And, in a moment...you notice yourself on a path in a valley...with grassy fields on both sides...and there is a hill you notice in front of you...with a hill top that is shining bright because of the Sunshine...

Pause

You...continue to walk on the path...as you continue to enjoy the surroundings and how you feel looking at all the scenic beauty...perhaps there is a water stream somewhere...the gorgeous trees, the fragrance of moss and flowers, butterflies on the bushes, and birds in the trees...hopping from one branch to another...

You notice the natural beauty and you keep walking forward...

And as you walk...you do feel...and you feel tired...and you wonder what makes you feel tired...

Longer Pause

And as you think about what makes you feel tired...you notice your coat...and you are perhaps feeling tired because of the old rugged coat that you have on...which makes you feel tired and you are unable to walk fast...it drags you down...it makes you tired...

And I wonder why...

Pause

As you look at your coat, you notice that it is old with many pockets...two front pockets and two side pockets...and they are full of some old stuff and clutter...

And you want to reach the hill top to enjoy the birds eye view of the valley...you want to reach the top, the ideal top, the goal is to be there...to be at your ideal weight...

And, I know you can do it...because everybody can...

Pause

You put your hands inside the pockets…and you notice…old papers and stones with many things written on them…that people may have told you knowingly or unknowingly and caused you emotional pain…

And because you have been carrying these in your coat….it makes you feel heavy and tired…and you can barely move forward…

Pause

You know you cannot let your past drive your present…it cannot make you feel heavy, fat, and tired…

The time has come to get rid of the coat now.

Longer Pause

And, I wonder if you can discard the coat somewhere in your valley before you move forward and reach the hill top…

Longer Pause

You have gotten rid of the old heavy rugged coat...and as soon as you have taken if off...you feel free...

You feel light...and energetic...

You are excited to reach the hill top by running towards it...

So....run and reach the hill top...that's your goal...and you can achieve any goal if you feel happy, energetic, and free from the past...

Longer Pause

In a moment you see yourself on the hill top...as someone who is freer, lighter, and happier...

That's right...

Ego Strengthening Script

And as you continue to listen to me and allow yourself to be more receptive and continue to drift deeper and deeper...

You have decided and are fully ready to make significant changes to your body and life to make it even happier and fulfilling.

Pause

And with every word you hear, you become fully aware of the times in the past that made you feel confident and good about yourself. This could be a time from teenage or yearly adulthood...

Get the knowing of that time now...

And as you think about those situations, I wonder if you can choose one that made you feel amazing, happy, confident, and made you believe in your worth.

Longer Pause

And, now that you think of that incident...I want you to watch it in your mind...and as you begin to watch it...you begin to watch it from the beginning...from the time the incident started...

And knowing what you did and how it made you feel and what all it made you think about yourself...

Become aware of those positive emotions and thoughts now...

That's right.

Longer Pause

And now you come to the end of it...

The time has come to watch it on a big TV screen...or even bigger...perhaps a projector screen in a room.

And, I wonder if you can imagine watching that good event...which made you feel great

about yourself...made you feel confident, happy, and proud...
Imagine that incident being played on a big projector screen and you are sitting on a couch watching it...

You have its controller in your hand...with many buttons on it...

And as you begin to watch it...you increase the volume to the level of 10...

That's right...

And as you continue to watch...you reach that moment which gave you maximum happiness and confidence...

And as you reach there...you zoom in the scene 10 times...

That's right...

Pause

And you can make the colours brighter and vivid...

Its loud, clear, and vivid....

And you take a mental screenshot of this....and store it somewhere in your mind...

Find a place in your mind to keep the screenshot saved.

Longer Pause

And, you know the place where you have stored it...and every time you feel low in life, you simply remind yourself of all the confidence and happiness your past self had achieved...and you can achieve it again...you can show this screenshot to empower your present self...

Longer Pause

And I wonder if you can practice everyday filling yourself with the color of confidence as soon as you wake up...to feel great in the morning and stay with the feeling throughout the day...

So, imagine a color of confidence...that you resonate with...it is different for everyone...

Think of a color that relates to confidence for you.

Pause

And slowly and slowly allow that colour to move into your body from all sides...perhaps starting from head or feet...

Let the colour reach every part of your body, fibre, cell, and bone...

Fill yourself up with the colour of confidence...the confidence that makes you feel happier, energetic, joyful, and positive.

With happiness and confidence, you can achieve your ideal goal weight...it just gets so much easier when you believe in yourself and have high self-esteem and self-worth...

Pause
You know that you have been confident before and you are confident and get even

more confident when you practice filling yourself up with the colour of confidence every morning...

The more your practice it the stronger your confidence becomes...

You lose weight when you eat right and exercise to burn off extra calories. This confidence helps you gain control on your eating habits and how you live your life...

And with every passing day, you notice your confidence goes to the next level...

With high level of confidence, it gets easier for you to know the ways to achieve your goal weight. And, with every passing day, your self-esteem and self-worth is increasing....

You think and talk confidently...and its visible in your body language...you exude self confidence in your walk and how you behave with people...your friends and family are amazed to see you talk so confidently...

Longer Pause

You allow yourself to release all the fears and other negative emotions...that serve no purpose...and allow yourself to feel the positive emotions like security, freedom, positivity, happiness, confidence, calmness...contentment...

Pause

You are aligned and centred at all times... always looking at living your present day and living it mindfully to achieve the daily goals...living each day beautifully and productively.

Longer Pause

You maintain calm and relaxed...focused and mindful. You are confident and secure about everything.

Pause

More Weight Loss

And as you continue to listen to each word I say and allow yourself to go deeper and deeper into a beautiful state of relaxation...

You are open to all my suggestions and this audio is designed to keep weight off permanently...so that you become lean, slim, happy, and even more positive person.

Pause

As you listen to this audio, you are reconditioning your mind to become a new person with a leaner and slimmer body having new eating habits.

With new eating habits, you feel empowered and happier and perhaps become a role model for others...by setting such great example.

Pause

You enjoy life and eat only when you are physical hungry and you eat to nurture and nourish your body...and no other time, you eat food.

In the past, you ate more than your body needed and perhaps you ate to satiate your emotional and mental needs. And because you ate more than what was required, you stored this extra energy as fat.

Pause

To burn this extra stored fat, you eat less each day and when you eat less that you require for the storage will make up the difference.

Longer Pause

And, because your stomach is now restricted, you will naturally eat lesser amounts of food and burn the fat faster. And, whatever healthy foods you will eat, you will be able to satisfy your hunger. You eat less and burn fat faster.

When you eat lesser amounts of healthy food, it shows up on your body and face. Your become slimmer and leaner with every passing day and you are amused to see the clothes getting lose on you.

Pause

You look forward to wearing fitter and smarter clothes and this motivates you even more to exercise and eat less.

You are consistently eating lesser amounts of food because your stomach is now shrunken to a size of a golf ball.

And because of this, you eat much lesser portions of food...and you see yourself as more confident person. You are happy with this transformation and your new form.

Pause

And I wonder if you allow these suggestions to sink into your subconscious for the purpose of your highest good. Also...you notice an image of your future slimmer self-flashing in your mind, the self who enjoys eating lesser amounts of nutritious and healthy food.

Longer Pause

And you have a changed mindset now...the mindset that you have enough to eat and you will never be starved. And, because there is plenty of food around you, you eat it when you want to it and how much you want to eat it. You will not hoard food inside you that makes you fat.

You are losing weight faster every day as you make a conscious effort to eat less because you know that your stomach is a size of a golf ball.

Pause

And as you continue to eat lesser amounts of food, you see yourself slimming down and getting into the shape that you desire. The excess weight is coming off...perhaps melting away...and vanishing...

That's right.

You are in complete control of your life...and your eating habits.

Weight Loss – Object of Past

And you continue to listen to me because you have a wonderful goal in your mind to be at your ideal goal weight...

You know that your stomach is now of a golf ball size and can take in much lesser amounts of foods...

And you are excited to achieve the weight loss results because of the gastric band fitted on your stomach...

Pause

You want to achieve you ideal goal weight and when you think every day about your weight, you must only think of it as the thing of past...and the goal of this recording is to help you let go of the weight problem so that your powerful subconscious mind can keep you focused on the road of weight loss for you to achieve a much slimmer and fitter body...looking absolutely stunning and attractive.

That's right…

Pause

And, I wonder if you can think of your weight issue as an object…it could be anything that comes to your mind…

Think of it as an object…and the object is a depiction of not only your weight, the pounds or kilos but also all the causes that led you to gain weight…the old habits of eating excess food and unhealthy food or eating when you were emotionally hungry…

Longer Pause

And all the effects of being overweight…think of all those and see the causes and effects in the object…

And, I wonder if you could give it a color…

And a texture….

Perhaps observe the shape of the object…

And get the knowing of its weight…is it too heavy?

Get the knowing of how this heavy object has made you feel about yourself in the past…

And now imagine what if you did not have to carry this object…how would your life be different?

Longer Pause

So, you now the time has come to put the weight problem down…put the object down…

And as soon as you do that…you feel the sense of calm all around you…and inside of you…

You can notice all the causes and effects of your old weight issue in that object and the time has come to let go of it completely…because it's not solving any purpose…

And you imagine seeing a helium balloon coming down to take this object with it…far away…away from you…away from your body…

The helium balloon comes down with every breath you take and with every word I say…becoming bigger and bigger as it comes closer and closer…

Longer Pause

And in a moment, you notice the balloon attaching itself to the object magically and takes a flight back to the sky with the object…attached to it…

That's right…

You notice it going up and up…far away…and you notice it becoming smaller and smaller because its moving farther and farther away…back to the sky…across the sky…

And as that happens…you start to feel so much lighter…and freer…as you have completely removed the object of weight from your life…

And you can time travel in your future and see how you look six months from now with the gastric band fitted on your stomach...with no weight object...eating healthily and exercising daily...

That's right...

Meet your future self now...and see how your future self greets and meets you...welcoming and accepting...

And, I wonder if you can move into the body of your future self to feel it and feel how your future self feels and thinks at the ideal goal weight...

And as you enter the body of your future self... you can feel the self's strong, slender, and attractive body...

Pause

See what clothes the future self is wearing...

Notice how the future self is talking and walking...is it more confident?

Now, have a heart to heart conversation with the future self and ask for advice and words of wisdom...perhaps the future self has something amazing to share with you that will change your life for good...

Ask what you need to know the most...and you will get all the guidance from your wise future self...

Longer Pause

Make a mental note of the advice and guidance given by the future self..

And with that...you know that the object of weight has gone far away and can never return...all the causes leading to weight gain and the effects have been dissolved...

You can visit your future self anytime and ask for the guidance or just simply meet by closing your eyes and counting down from 10 down to 0...and at 0..you can imagine your future self...

You can do that...anytime to feel motivated to stay on the road to weight loss...and to seek guidance...

That's right...

Reinforcement Script

As you continue to listen to me...and as we tap into your very powerful mind...you are going to have an amazing relationship with yourself...

You are going to understand yourself and your body better...

You will have a changed and better relationship with food...

Pause

You allow yourself to open to only positive thoughts and be absolutely closed to old negative thoughts, beliefs, and negative emotions...arising from past events...

You are in control...the more control you are...the better is your state of mind...with more control... you feel more relaxed...

That's right...

And I wonder if you can imagine yourself standing on top of a staircase and this time...you see yourself a little different...

You see yourself as more in control...feeling calm and relaxed...knowing all your positive qualities and strengths...

Longer Pause

And perhaps at your ideal goal weight...

Get the sense of it...notice how you look, feel, and how you are standing with straight body posture exuding unending confidence.

I am going to count down from 10 down to 0...it reinforces that this is you. Confident, at your ideal goal weight, knowing all your positive qualities...

10...stepping down the staircase

9...

8....

7...strengthening this is you...

6...

5...

4...knowing this is you

3...confident

2...sealing in the image in your subconscious

1...

0...This is You.

You now begin to think of all the reasons you want to lose weight...and the benefits attached to being at the ideal goal weight...

Longer Pause

Perhaps some of the benefits are more energy, good health, fitter and slimmer, feel attractive, more in control, and wear attractive and fashionable clothes...

Maybe you would be more active and energetic...have better sex life...

The list goes on...

Pause

Your subconscious mind which is the powerful and creative mind will find many healthy and creative ways to move your body more...and with every passing day...you are becoming more and more comfortable with the new body image...at your ideal goal weight...With every passing moment... the fact is strengthening that you have achieved your ideal goal weight...and you are well aware of what that brings with it...all the happiness.. Your drive and motivation is to feel happier every day.

Pause

You may find that that your body and mind are harmoniously working together to help you achieve your ideal goal weight...

That's right.

You are more ready than ever to live a fulfilling life...to be aware and conscious of all the good things that life has to offer to you...

Pause

You begin to realize that you can be relaxed and calm...and are in flow with everything that is happening around you...

With every passing day...you are more energetic and more productive...

That's right...

Affirmations

1. You are in control of how much you eat (7 seconds pause)
2. You deserve to feel happy and look great (7 seconds pause)
3. You enjoy exercising (7 seconds pause)
4. You eat only when you are hungry (7 seconds pause)
5. You are getting slimmer every day (7 seconds pause)
6. You choose to eat right (7 seconds pause)
7. You deserve to be healthier and attractive (7 seconds pause)
8. You love your body and care for it (7 seconds pause)
9. You are developing healthy eating habits (7 seconds pause)
10. You are happy exercising (7 seconds pause)
11. You are reaching your ideal goal weight soon (7 seconds pause)

12. You eat smaller portions (7 seconds pause)
13. You drink 8 to 10 glasses of water everyday (7 seconds pause)
14. You eat fruits and vegetables and enjoy eating them (7 seconds pause)
15. You celebrate your life and healthy choices (7 seconds pause)
16. You have a flat stomach (7 seconds pause)
17. You are getting attractive and even more charming with every passing day (7 seconds pause)
18. You take charge of your life and body (7 seconds pause)
19. You fall asleep every night effortlessly (7 seconds pause)
20. You love and appreciate your body (7 seconds pause)
21. You love changing your body (7 seconds pause)
22. Your metabolism is faster than before (7 seconds pause)
23. You are mindful and live every moment (7 seconds pause)

24. You are lovable (7 seconds pause)
25. You are a beautiful person (7 seconds pause)
26. You love yourself unconditionally (7 seconds pause)
27. You are complete and whole. (7 seconds pause)
28. You are confident and courageous (7 seconds pause)
29. You forgive yourself for all the past mistakes (7 seconds pause)
30. You stay in present and are more mindful (7 seconds pause)
31. You are confident (7 seconds pause)
32. You have high self-esteem (7 seconds pause)
33. You are losing weight every day (7 seconds pause)
34. You are focused on your weight loss journey (7 seconds pause)
35. You pay attention to your food intake (7 seconds pause)
36. You chew your food many times (7 seconds pause)

37. You maintain sleep hygiene (7 seconds pause)
38. You love yourself unconditionally (7 seconds pause)
39. Your body is getting fitter and slimmer (7 seconds pause)
40. You are successful (7 seconds pause)
41. You are confident and motivated (7 seconds pause)
42. You believe in yourself (7 seconds pause)
43. You are good enough (7 seconds pause)
44. You enjoy healthy foods (7 seconds pause)
45. You do pleasurable activities everyday (7 seconds pause)
46. You are intelligent and wise (7 seconds pause)
47. You are lovable, open to receive and give love (7 seconds pause)
48. You enjoy your life (7 seconds pause)
49. You enjoy healthy food (7 seconds pause)

50. You have a beautiful relationship with food and your body (7 seconds pause)
51. You have a lot of love and approval for yourself. (7 seconds pause)
52. You are at peace with yourself in your body, heart and soul. (7 seconds pause)
53. As each day passes, you feel that you are healthier and stronger inside. (7 seconds pause)
54. Every day, you are learning how to love and appreciate your body. (7 seconds pause)
55. Being yourself is the safest way for you to be. (7 seconds pause)
56. You focus on all the good that is happening in your life. (7 seconds pause)
57. It becomes easier and easier for you to trust your body. (7 seconds pause)
58. You can feel your body and mind getting healed. (7 seconds pause)
59. You are choosing to take in breaths of relaxation and breathe out all your stress. (7 seconds pause)

60. Your health and your life are moving in the direction of improvement. (7 seconds pause)
61. A healing white light surrounds you and is protecting you. (7 seconds pause)
62. Your entire food intake is nourishing your body and healing it well. (7 seconds pause)
63. Every baby step you take is getting you closer to your ideal goal weight. (7 seconds pause)
64. You progress comes above any perfection for you. (7 seconds pause)
65. Your intuition is your guiding light and helps you decide what to eat and how to live your life. (7 seconds pause)
66. You are naturally connecting with like-minded people who bring in positivity. (7 seconds pause)
67. It is best for you to let go of your past. Letting go of the past is safe for you now. (7 seconds pause)
68. You can feel the beginning of changes in everything around you. (7 seconds pause)

69. You are now focused, determined and healthy. (7 seconds pause)
70. You choose for yourself to be slim and healthy. (7 seconds pause)
71. You can see new doors opening in your life with a lot of new and exciting things. (7 seconds pause)
72. You have the ability to heal your body. You are healing your body. (7 seconds pause)
73. You can do this and so you are doing this. Your body is healing right now. (7 seconds pause)
74. A higher power is guiding you along your way. (7 seconds pause)
75. You are a strong, energetic person. (7 seconds pause)
76. You choose to see the best in everyone and so do they. (7 seconds pause)
77. You have faith in your ability of self-love. (7 seconds pause)
78. You truly love yourself for however you are. (7 seconds pause)
79. You have accepted and acknowledged your body shape and the beauty hidden in it.

80. You are the creator of your future. (7 seconds pause)
81. You have now moved on from the unhealthy, unhelpful behavioral pattern around food. (7 seconds pause)
82. The choices and decisions you make for yourself are for your higher good. (7 seconds pause)
83. You are no longer holding on to any regrets or guilt about your past food choices. (7 seconds pause)
84. You have accepted your body's shape and you feel blessed for what you have. (7 seconds pause)
85. You have moved farther away from relationships that don't contribute to your betterment. (7 seconds pause)
86. You acknowledge your own greatness. (7 seconds pause)
87. You allow yourself to feel good about being you. (7 seconds pause)
88. You have an acceptance for yourself. (7 seconds pause)
89. You are letting in the qualities of love in your heart. (7 seconds pause)

90. You see your future filled with hope and certainty. (7 seconds pause)
91. You find gratefulness in your heart for your body and all you do for your well-being. (7 seconds pause)
92. You indulge in a healthy amount of exercise on a regular basis. (7 seconds pause)
93. Your body is getting all the nutrients that it requires. (7 seconds pause)
94. You are developing a strong urge to eat food that is nutritious (7 seconds pause)
95. You feel good about yourself. (7 seconds pause)
96. You are on your way to attaining and maintaining your ideal weight. (7 seconds pause)
97. You are a strong, healthy person. (7 seconds pause)
98. You are now peaceful and calm. (7 seconds pause)
99. The Universe has gifted you with your mind, body and soul. (7 seconds pause)
100. Your body is your temple.

101.   You love your body and take care of it every single day.. (7 seconds pause)

Waking Up

In a moment, I am going to count you up from 1 to 5, and with each count up, you will slowly and gradually come back to the here and now.

Starting now

At 1...become aware of your breaths

2...start coming up

3...further up

4...all your spiritual, mental, emotional, physical bodies aligned...

5...feel the clothes on your body...eyes open wide awake.